Happiness Guide

How to boost your serotonin level

PV Mihalache

This book is for you my dear friend and I hope you will find advice and the answers to your questions.

I have to congratulate you for your choice, for having the courage to change your life and be happy!

Serotonin (5-hydroxytryptamine, 5-HT) is a monoamine neurotransmitter although some consider the chemical to be a hormone and act as a mood stabilizer helping to produce healthy sleeping patterns and is popularly thought to be a contributor of feelings of well-being and happiness.

"If you want to be happy, be." – Leo Tolstoy

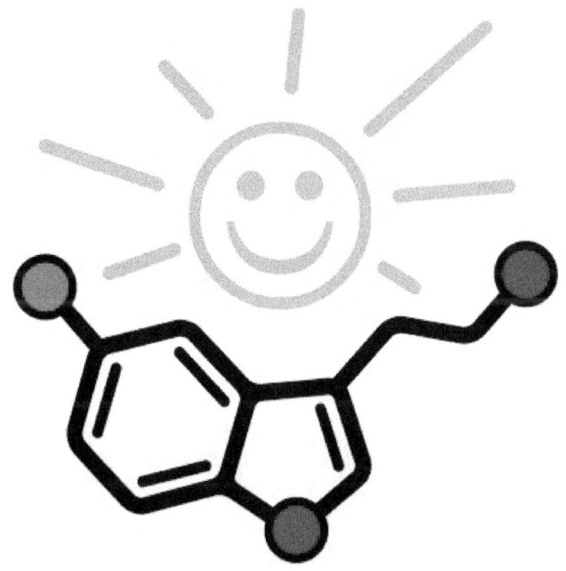

"Happiness is not something ready made. It comes from your own actions."~Dalai Lama

What is Serotonin?

Serotonin (5-hydroxytryptamine,5-HT) is a monoamine neurotransmitter although some consider the chemical to be a hormone and act as a mood stabilizer helping to produce healthy sleeping patterns and is popularly thought to be a contributor of feelings of well-being and happiness.

Serotonin acts as a neurotransmitter, a type of chemical that helps relay signals from one area of the brain to another. Although serotonin is manufactured in the brain, where it performs its primary functions, some 90% of our serotonin supply is found in the digestive tract and in blood platelets.

Biochemically derived from tryptophan*, serotonin is primarily found in the Gastro-Intestinal tract (GI tract), blood platelets and the Central Nervous System (CNS).

The 90% of the human body's total serotonin is located in the enterochromaffin cells in the GI tract, where it is used to regulate intestinal movements.

The reminder is synthesized in the serotonergic neurons of the Central Nervous System, where it has various functions. These include the regulation of mood, appetite and sleep. Serotonin also has some cognitive functions, including memory and learning .Modulations of serotonin at synapses is thought to be a major action of several classes of pharmacological antidepressants.

* Tryptophan is one of the 22 standard amino-acids and an essential amino-acid in the human diet.

Serotonin secreted from the enterochromaffin cells eventually finds its way out of tissues into the blood.

There, it is actively taken up by blood platelets, which store it.

When the platelets bind to a clot, they release serotonin, where it serves as a vasoconstrictor and helps to regulate homeostasis and blood clotting.

Serotonin also is a growth factor for some types of cells, which may give it a role in wound healing.

In mice and humans, alterations in serotonin levels and signaling have been shown to regulate bone mass.#

In humans, increased blood serotonin levels have been shown to be significant negative predictor of low bone density.

Since serotonin signals resource availability it is not surprising that it affects organ development.

Many human studies have shown that nutrition in early life can influence, in adulthood, such things as body fatness, blood lipids, blood pressure, atherosclerosis, behaviour learning and longevity.

Serotonin is thought to be especially active in constricting smooth muscles, transmitting impulses between nerve cells, regulating cyclic body processes and is regarded by some researchers as a chemical that is responsible for maintaining mood balance and that a deficit of serotonin leads to depression.

Because cannot cross the blood-brain barrier, serotonin that is used inside the brain must be produced within it via a unique biochemical conversion process.

It begins with tryptophan, a building block to proteins.

Cells that make serotonin use trypophan hydroxylase, a chemical reactor which, when combined with tryptophan , forms 5-hydroxytryptamine, otherwise known as Serotonin.

What role does serotonin play in our health?

As a neurotransmitter, serotonin helps to relay messages from one area of the brain to another.

Because of the widespread distribution of its cells, it is believed to influence a variety of psychological and other body functions.

Of the approximately 40 million brain cells, most are influenced either directly or indirectly by serotonin. This includes brain cells related to mood, sexual desire and function, appetite, sleep, memory and learning, temperature regulation, and some social behaviour.

In terms of our body function, serotonin can also affect the functioning of our cardiovascular system, muscles, and various elements in the endocrine system.

Researchers have also found evidence that serotonin may play a role in regulating milk production in the breast, and that a defect within the serotonin network may be one underlying cause of SIDS (sudden infant death syndrome).

Serotonin influences both directly and indirectly the majority of brain cells.

The following is a list of things that it is thought that serotonin could affect:

- **Bowel function.** Most of the body's serotonin is found in the gastrointestinal tract where it regulates bowel function and movements. It also plays a part in reducing the appetite while consuming a meal.

- **Mood**. It is most well known for its role in the brain where it plays a major part in mood, anxiety and happiness. Illicit mood-altering drugs such as Ecstasy and LSD cause a massive rise in serotonin levels.
- **Clotting**. Its third major role is in the formation of blood clots. Serotonin is released by platelets when there is a wound, and the resulting vasoconstriction (narrowing of the tiny arteries - arterioles) reduces blood flow and aids the formation of blood clots.
- **Nausea**. If you eat something that is toxic or irritating, more serotonin is produced in the gut to increase transit time and expel the irritant in diarrhoea. This increase in blood serotonin levels also causes nausea by stimulating the nausea area in the brain.
- **Bone density**. Studies have shown that a persistent high level of serotonin in the bones can lead to an increase in osteoporosis.
- **Sexual function**. Low serotonin levels in the intoxicated state are thought to contribute to the associated increase in libido, while those taking medication that increase serotonin levels are seen to have a reduction in libido and sexual function.

The most widely distributed , and the most widely studied, neurotransmitter in the brain, serotonin regulates a vast range of psychological and biological functions, including mood, sleep, arousal and appetite.

Many people think of serotonin as nature's "feel-good" chemical.

Now, researchers at Cambridge University and UCLA have found that serotonin also plays a critical role in regulating emotions such as impulsive aggression during social decision making.

Impulsive aggression is the tendency to respond with hostility or aggression when faced with serious frustration.

The researchers believe their results suggest that serotonin plays a critical role in social decision making by normally keeping aggressive social responses in check.

By manipulating the diet, the researchers were able to lower serotonin levels in the brain of healthy volunteers. Tryptophan, the essential amino-acid necessary for the body to produce serotonin, can be obtained only through diet.

Twenty healthy volunteers fasted overnight and were then given a protein drink, receiving drinks with tryptophan one day and without it the next.

On both days, the study participants played the "Ultimatum Game", in which one player poses a way to split a sum of money with a partner. If the partner accepts the offer, both players are paid accordingly. If the offer is rejected, however, neither player is paid.

Some of the offers were considered "fair" (45 percent of the cash) while others were considered "unfair" (18 percent of the cash).

When the players serotonin levels were low they showed increased aggression towards offers they perceived to be unfair.

The findings highlight why some people become aggressive or act impulsively when they have not eaten, says lead researcher Molly Crocket at the University of Cambridge Behavioural and Clinical Neuroscience Institute.

Because the body needs tryptophan to make serotonin, levels of the neurotransmitter naturally fluctuate throughout the day, depending on food intake. Food such as chocolate, oats, bananas and poultry, especially turkey, are rich in tryptophan.

"Tryptophan is an essential amino-acid, and you have to get it in your diet, which is not hard to do", says psychiatrist Emil Coccaro, an expert on impulsive aggression and mood disorders at the University of Chicago.

He notes that when someone is given a drink containing amino acids other than tryptophan, the liver pulls tryptophan from the blood to make the protein with the new amino acid the person was just given.

This process causes a drop in blood tryptophan level to about ten percent to twenty percent of what they are normally, leading to a reduction in the amount of newly made serotonin and , thus, a decrease in serotonin activity.

Under normal circumstances, serotonin works in the frontal areas of the brain to inhibit the firing of the amygdala, the almond-shaped structure that controls fear, anger and other emotional responses.

"If there is less serotonin in the frontal brain areas, there will be less inhibition on the amygdala," says Coccaro.

"When the amygdala is stimulated by outside novel and potentially threatening events, it will become more active, driving the person to act on their impulses.

People who suffer from mood disorders or impulsiveness caused by low serotonin levels can be treated with a class of drugs called selective serotonin reuptake inhibitors, or SSRIs, which enhance neurotransmission and make more serotonin available to nerve cells in the brain.

Although Crockett's study examined low serotonin levels in healthy people, she says she is not certain what the results of a similar study would be in people with disorders in which low serotonin levels are implicated, such as depression or obsessive compulsive disorder.

"It's possible that lowering serotonin would have a similar or perhaps even more extreme effect, since the system is probably more vulnerable in these individuals," she said in an e-mail. "On the other hand, it's equally plausible that tryptophan depletion would have a negligible effect since serotonin is already low and lowering it more may not change much in terms of behavioural output."

Is a link between serotonin and depression?

There are many researchers who believe that an imbalance in serotonin levels may influence mood in a way that leads to depression.

Possible problems include low brain cell production of serotonin, a lack of receptor sites able to receive the serotonin that is made, inability of serotonin to reach the receptor sites, or a shortage in tryptophan, the chemical from which serotonin is made.

If any of these biochemical glitches occur, researchers believe it can lead to depression, as well as obsessive-compulsive disorder, anxiety, panic, and even excess anger.

One theory about how depression develops centres on the regeneration of brain cells, a process that some believe is mediated by serotonin, and ongoing throughout our lives. According to Princeton neuroscientist Barry Jacobs, PhD, depression may occur when there is a suppression of new brain cells and that stress is the most important precipitator of depression. He believes that common antidepressant medications known as SSRIs, which are designed to boost serotonin levels, help kick off the production of new brain cells, which in turn allows the depression to lift.

Although it is widely believed that a serotonin deficiency plays a role in depression, there is no way to measure its levels in the living brain.

Therefore, there have not been any studies proving that brain levels of this or any neurotransmitter are in short supply when depression or any mental illness develops.

However, levels of serotonin in the blood *are* measurable and have been shown to be lower in people who suffer from depression. However, researchers still don't know if serotonin levels in the blood reflect levels in the brain. They also don't know whether the dip in serotonin causes the depression, or the depression causes serotonin levels to drop.

Antidepressant medications that work on serotonin levels - SSRIs (selective serotonin reuptake inhibitors) and SNRIs (serotonin and norepinephrine reuptake inhibitors) - are believed to reduce symptoms of depression, but exactly how they work is not yet fully understood.

Serotonin is known to be a critical stress hormone. It influences body temperature, blood pressure, clotting of blood, immunities, pain endurance, sleep, digestion, and circadian body rhythms. There are medical concerns that serotonin deficiency will increase the risk of behavioural problems such as aggression, depression, suicide, drug use, and hypersexual behaviours.

With serotonin affecting the overall mood, other aspects which stem from a less than happy feeling due to serotonin deficiencies are also involved.

Sleep disturbances are prevalent among people suffering from depression. Increasing serotonin levels will rectify such insomniatic disorders.

Emotional eating is also related to depression and lack of serotonin levels. Binge eating and carbohydrate cravings will lead to undesired weight gain. Generally, overweight people prove to have a well below normal serotonin level. In certain clinical trials, elevating brain serotonin levels reduces calorie consumption in the obese with no apparent effort to do so. Replenishing serotonin levels normalizes eating behaviours by reducing carbohydrates and fats with the reduction of body weight as a result.

It is implied that serotonin is a key neurotransmitter to migraine headaches. Studies have proved that replenishing serotonin levels will relieve migraines and reduce the need for pain medications. The serotonin has the ability to relax the muscles and control the dilation of blood vessels.

Serotonin will calm the nervous system which will relieve tension and anxiety as a result. The stiffness, sleep disturbance, irritable bowel problems, and menstrual disorders which are associated with fibromyalgia will benefit from an enhancement of serotonin levels.

Depression and anxiety are strongly associated with asthmatic sufferers. There is a decrease in pulmonary control resulting in emergency room and doctor visits. Normal activities are sabotaged because of consistent breathing problems. Children with asthma are especially prone to depression due to the fact that they are purposely prevented from normal activities because of their condition.

Serotonin is abundantly found in the digestive system as well as the brain. When proper foods are digested, the body will produce natural serotonin.

There are several drugs available to treat depression caused by a chemical imbalance and serotonin deficiency. SSRI, selective serotonin reuptake inhibitors, are pills prescribed to increase the brain's serotonin levels by increasing the length that is stays in the brain. Unfortunately, these prescribed medications come with unwelcomed side effects such as nausea, irritability sexual dysfunction, and more.

Besides the prescription drugs available to enhance serotonin deficiency, there are also natural supplements which have a mood boosting effect as well. 5-HTP is known as the natural antidepressant.

There is evidence confirming that 5-hydroxytryptophan will reduce depression. There has been decades of studies to prove this theory.

Particular studies compared patients taking fluvoxamine, an SSRI, to those taking 5-HTP, a natural supplement.

The prescribed medication and the supplement were equally effective in relieving depression. However, the 5-HTP was far more tolerant and safe over the fluvoxamine since it had fewer side effects. If there were any adverse reaction, they were substantially less severe than the effects of the SSRI.

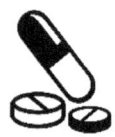

Can diet influence our supply of serotonin?

Serotonin is synthesized from the amino acid tryptophan. Many foods contain tryptophan, so the common belief is that by eating foods high in tryptophan, you can boost your serotonin levels.

The relationship between tryptophan and serotonin is part of what's commonly considered the food-mood connection.

Serotonin isn't found in foods, but tryptophan is. Foods high in protein, iron, riboflavin, and vitamin B6 all tend to contain large amounts of the amino acid. Unfortunately, though, boosting your serotonin levels isn't as simple as eating a "high tryptophan diet."

The tryptophan you find in food has to compete with other amino acids to be absorbed into the brain, so it's unlikely to have much of an effect on your serotonin levels. This differs from tryptophan supplements, which contain purified tryptophan and do have an effect on serotonin levels.

Unlike calcium-rich foods, which can directly increase your blood levels of this mineral, there are no foods that can directly increase your body's supply of serotonin. That said, there are foods and some nutrients that can increase levels of tryptophan, the amino acid from which serotonin is made.

Protein-rich foods, such as meat or chicken, contain high levels of tryptophan. Tryptophan appears in dairy foods, nuts, and fowl.

Ironically, however, levels of both tryptophan and serotonin drop after eating a meal packed with protein. Why? According to nutritionist Elizabeth Somer, when you eat a high-protein meal, you "flood the blood with both tryptophan and its competing amino acids," all fighting for entry into the brain.

That means only a small amount of tryptophan gets through and serotonin levels don't rise.

But eat a carbohydrate-rich meal, and your body triggers a release of insulin. This, Somer says, causes any amino acids in the blood to be absorbed into the body, but not the brain. Except for, you guessed it ,tryptophan!

It remains in the bloodstream at high levels following a carbohydrate meal, which means it can freely enter the brain and cause serotonin levels to rise, she says.

What can also help: Getting an adequate supply of vitamin B-6, which can influence the rate at which tryptophan is converted to serotonin.

Here's a brief explanation of the mechanism behind the effect of food on serotonin levels: after consumption of a carbohydrate-rich meal, the hormone insulin is secreted. Insulin lowers the blood levels of most amino acids (the building blocks of protein), except for tryptophan.

Amino acids compete for transportation across the blood-brain barrier, and when there is a larger proportion of tryptophan, it enters the brain at a higher rate, thus boosting serotonin production.

To make matters more interesting, tryptophan is present in many protein-rich foods, which have been found to prevent serotonin production. So, you can see how intricate and complex this system is.

In terms of the effects of actual foods on serotonin, here are some suggestions from nutritionists:

- If you're having trouble falling asleep, try a small snack of carbohydrate-rich food. Warm milk may work for the psychological comfort, but also because milk contains a moderate amount of carbohydrate in the form of lactose (milk sugar).
- If you tend to have only carbohydrates (bread, plain bagel or muffin) before class, and you often fall asleep during class, try adding some protein by putting some hard cheese (soft cheese, cheddar, American, Swiss, etc.) or peanut butter on the bagel. Or, have a yogurt or cottage cheese instead.
- For those who are active (athletes or exercisers), don't be fooled by carbohydrate's relaxing effects. You'll do best with a diet rich in grains/starches, legumes (dried beans and peas), fruit, and vegetables in order to get carbohydrates for muscle energy. Don't skimp on protein either, which is necessary for muscle growth and repair. Additionally, include some fat for satiety and healthy skin.

The carbohydrate/tryptophan/serotonin pathway is simply a hypothesis at this point. Since each of us is unique, in order to get a "desired effect" from food, you would need to experiment eating different foods and observing how your body reacts to each of them.

You'll also need to take into consideration your other lifestyle choices, how much sleep you get, whether or not you exercise regularly, the medications you take, your stress levels, when figuring out what affects your moods in what manners.

Attention span difficulties may or may not be attributed to what you consume. Many college students go for long periods of time without eating. This certainly can affect your concentration.

Our brains need glucose, and if we deny it through lack of food, our bodies have to work harder to break down stored carbohydrates for glucose that'll be used to feed our brain and central nervous system.

That's why it's a good idea to have something to eat about every four hours or so. Be prepared by carrying some snacks with you, especially if you're busy and short on time.

Some portable snack ideas include fruit, low-fat granola bars, nuts, and low-fat crackers.

Food with a high percentage of carbs will help build up your tryptophan.

There's a reason why foods like mac and cheese and mashed potatoes are considered "comfort foods," especially when the weather is dreary.

While high-tryptophan foods won't boost serotonin on their own, there is one possible cheat to this system: carbs.

It's possible that eating foods high in tryptophan with a healthy serving of carbohydrates can have an effect on your serotonin levels.

When you eat carbs, more insulin is released into your system. Insulin promotes the absorption of amino acids into the heart, muscles, and organs. The tryptophan left behind now makes up a larger portion of the blood's amino acid "pool," meaning that it's more likely that it will be absorbed through the brain barrier.

While they can't compete with supplements, which you should not be taking without approval from your doctor, the foods listed below contain high amounts of tryptophan. Your best chance at achieving a serotonin boost without using supplements is to eat them often, with a serving of healthy carbohydrates, like rice, oatmeal, or whole-grain bread.

Can exercise boost serotonin levels?

Exercise can do a lot to improve your mood, and across the board, studies have shown that regular exercise can be as effective a treatment for depression as antidepressant medication orpsychotherapy.

In the past, it was believed that several weeks of working out was necessary to see the effects on depression, but new research conducted at the University of Texas at Austin found that just a single 40-minute period of exercise can have an immediate effect on mood.

That said, it remains unclear of the exact mechanism by which exercise accomplishes this. While some believe it affects serotonin levels, to date there are no definitive studies showing that this is the case.

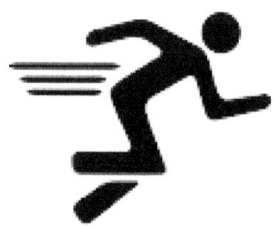

Do men and women have the same amount of serotonin?

Do men and women have the same amount of serotonin, and does it act the same way in their brain and body?

Studies show that men do have slightly more serotonin than women, but the difference is thought to be negligible.

Interestingly, however, a study published in September 2007 in the journal *Biological Psychiatry* showed there might be a huge difference in how men and women react to a reduction in serotonin -- and that may be one reason why women suffer from depression far more than men.

Using a technique called "tryptophan depletion," which reduces serotonin levels in the brain, researchers found that men became impulsive but not necessarily depressed.

Women, on the other hand, experienced a marked drop in mood and became more cautious, an emotional response commonly associated with depression.

While the serotonin processing system seems the same in both sexes, researchers now believe men and women may use serotonin differently.

Although studies are still in their infancy, researchers say defining these differences may be the beginning of learning why more women than men experience anxiety and mood disorders, while more men experience alcoholism, ADHS and impulse control disorders.

There is also some evidence that female hormones may also interact with serotonin to cause some symptoms to occur or worsen during the premenstrual time, during the postpartum period, or around the time of menopause.

Not coincidentally, these are all periods when sex hormones are in flux. Men, on the other hand, generally experience a steady level of sex hormones until middle age, when the decline is gradual.

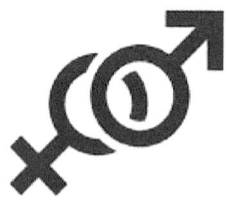

Serotonin and brain-related condition

Since both dementia and Alzheimer's disease are brain-related conditions, does serotonin play a role in either problem?

The word dementia describes a set of symptoms that may include memory loss and difficulties with thinking, problem-solving or language. Dementia is caused when the brain is damaged by diseases, such as Alzheimer's disease or a series of strokes.

Alzheimer's disease is the most common cause of dementia. The word dementia describes a set of symptoms that can include memory loss and difficulties with thinking, problem-solving or language.

These symptoms occur when the brain is damaged by certain diseases, including Alzheimer's disease.

Alzheimer's disease, named after the doctor who first described it (Alois Alzheimer), is a physical disease that affects the brain.

During the course of the disease, proteins build up in the brain to form structures called 'plaques' and 'tangles'.

This leads to the loss of connections between nerve cells, and eventually to the death of nerve cells and loss of brain tissue.

People with Alzheimer's also have a shortage of some important chemicals in their brain. These chemical messengers help to transmit signals around the brain.

When there is a shortage of them, the signals are not transmitted as effectively. As discussed below, current treatments for Alzheimer's disease can help boost the levels of chemical messengers in the brain, which can help with some of the symptoms.

Alzheimer's is a progressive disease. This means that gradually, over time, more parts of the brain are damaged. As this happens, more symptoms develop. They also become more severe.

In much the same way that we lose bone mass as we age, some researchers believe that the activity of neurotransmitters also slows down as part of the aging process.

In one international study published in 2006, doctors from several research centres around the world noted a serotonin deficiency in brains of deceased Alzheimer's patients.

They hypothesized that the deficiency was because of a reduction in receptor sites -- cells capable of receiving transmissions of serotonin -- and that this in turn may be responsible for at least some of the memory-related symptoms of Alzheimer's disease.

There is no evidence to show that increasing levels of serotonin will prevent Alzheimer's disease or delay the onset or progression of dementia. However, as research into this area continues, this could also change.

What is serotonin syndrome?

Too little serotonin in the brain is thought to play a role in depression. Too much, however, can lead to excessive nerve cell activity, causing a potentially deadly collection of symptoms known as serotonin syndrome.

SSRI antidepressants are generally considered safe. However, a rare side effect of SSRIs called serotonin syndrome can occur when levels of this neuro-chemical in the brain rise too high.

Serotonin syndrome symptoms often begin within hours of taking a new medication that affects serotonin levels or excessively increasing the dose of one you are already taking.

-Symptoms may include:
-Confusion
-Agitation or restlessness
-Dilated pupils
-Headache
-Changes in blood pressure and/or temperature
-Nausea and/or vomiting
-Diarrhoea
-Rapid heart rate
-Tremor
-Loss of muscle coordination
-Twitching muscles
-Shivering and goose bumps
-Heavy sweating

In severe cases, serotonin syndrome can be life-threatening.

If you experience any of these symptoms, you or someone with you should seek medical attention immediately: high fever, seizures, irregular heartbeat, unconsciousness.

Serotonin syndrome can occur if you are taking medications, particularly antidepressants, that affect the body's level of serotonin.

The greatest risk of serotonin syndrome occurs if you are taking two or more drugs and/or supplements together that influence serotonin. For example you take a category of migraine medicines called triptans at the same tame you are taking an SSRI drug for depression, the end result can be a serotonin overload.

Problems are most likely to occur when you first start a medication or increase the dosage. Problems can also occur if you combine the older depression medications (known as MAOIs) with SSRIs.

The most commonly prescribed class of antidepressants , which work by increasing serotonin, are the serotonin reuptake inhibitors (SSRIs).

Other prescription and over-the-counter drugs that can raise serotonin levels alone or in combination to cause serotonin syndrome include: Serotonin and norepinephrine reuptake inhibitors (SNRIs), a class of antidepressants, Monoamine oxidase inhibitors (MAOIs), a class of antidepressants , certain medications prescribed for nausea.

Finally, recreational drugs such as ecstasy or LSD have also been linked to serotonin syndrome.

How to increase serotonin level ?

This will be the main part of the book and will show ways to increase the serotonin level and have a healthy lifestyle in a try to be happy.

It is more likely that the serotonin will be synthesised at a higher rate if we have a stress less life and we spend time with the ones we love and care about. Also diet, food and intake helps improve the level of serotonin.

In a classic study, those in the lowest quartile for positive emotions, died on average 10 years earlier than those in the highest quartile. Even taking into account possible confounders, other studies found the same solid link between feeling good and living longer.

In a series of recent studies, negative emotions were associated with increased disability due to mental and physical disorders, increased incidence of depression, increased suicide and increased mortality up to two decades later.

Positive emotions protected against these outcomes. A recent review including meta-analyses assessed cross-sectional, longitudinal and experimental studies and concluded that happiness is associated with and precedes numerous successful outcomes. Mood may influence social behaviour, and social support is one of the most studied psychosocial factors in relation to health and disease. Low social support is associated with higher levels of stress, depression, dysthymia and post traumatic stress disorder and with increased morbidity and mortality from a host of medical illnesses.

Serotonin may be associated with physical health as well as mood. In otherwise healthy individuals, a low prolactin response to the serotonin-releasing drug fenfluramine was associated with the metabolic syndrome, a risk factor for heart disease, suggesting that low serotonin may predispose healthy individuals to suboptimal physical as well as mental functioning.

Non pharmacological methods of raising brain serotonin may not only improve mood and social functioning of healthy people, a worthwhile objective even without additional considerations, but would also make it possible to test the idea that increases in brain serotonin may help protect against the onset of various mental and physical disorders.

Exposure to bright light is a possible approach to increasing serotonin without drugs. Bright light is, of course, a standard treatment for seasonal depression, but a few studies also suggest that it is an effective treatment for non seasonal depression and also reduces depressed mood in women with premenstrual dysphoric disorder and in pregnant women suffering from depression.

The evidence relating these effects to serotonin is indirect. In human postmortem brain, serotonin levels are higher in those who died in summer than in those who died in winter.

A similar conclusion came from a study on healthy volunteers, in which serotonin synthesis was assessed by measurements of the serotonin metabolite 5-hydroxyindoleacetic acid (5-HIAA) in the venous outflow from the brain.

There was also a positive correlation between serotonin synthesis and the hours of sunlight on the day the measurements were made, independent of season. In humans, there is certainly an interaction between bright light and the serotonin system. The mood-lowering effect of acute tryptophan depletion in healthy women is completely blocked by carrying out the study in bright light (3000 lux) instead of dim light.

Relatively few generations ago, most of the world population was involved in agriculture and was outdoors for much of the day. This would have resulted in high levels of bright light exposure even in winter. Even on a cloudy day, the light outside can be greater than 1000 lux, a level never normally achieved indoors. In a recent study carried out at around latitude 45° N, daily exposure to light greater than 1000 lux averaged about 30 minutes in winter and only about 90 minutes in summer among people working at least 30 hours weekly; weekends were included. In this group, summer bright light exposure was probably considerably less than the winter exposure of our agricultural ancestors. We may be living in a bright light-deprived society.

A large literature that is beyond the scope of this editorial exists on the beneficial effect of bright light exposure in healthy individuals. Lamps designed for the treatment of seasonal affective disorder, which provide more lux than is ever achieved by normal indoor lighting, are readily available, although incorporating their use into a daily routine may be a challenge for some. However, other strategies, both personal and institutional, exist.

Better use of daylight in buildings is an issue that architects are increasingly aware of. Working indoors does not have to be associated with suboptimal exposure to bright light.

Other strategy that may raise brain serotonin is exercise. A comprehensive review of the relation between exercise and mood concluded that antidepressant and anxiolytic effects have been clearly demonstrated.

In the United Kingdom the National Institute for Health and Clinical Excellence, which works on behalf of the National Health Service and makes recommendations on treatments according to the best available evidence, has published a guide on the treatment of depression. The guide recommends treating mild clinical depression with various strategies, including exercise rather than antidepressants, because the risk–benefit ratio is poor for antidepressant use in patients with mild depression.

Exercise improves mood in subclinical populations as well as in patients. The most consistent effect is seen when regular exercisers undertake aerobic exercise at a level with which they are familiar.

However, some scepticism remains about the antidepressant effect of exercise, and the National Institute of Mental Health in the United States is currently funding a clinical trial of the antidepressant effect of exercise that is designed to overcome sources of potential bias and threats to internal and external validity that have limited previous research.

Several lines of research suggest that exercise increases brain serotonin function in the human brain. Post and colleagues measured biogenic amine metabolites in cerebrospinal fluid (CSF) of patients with depression before and after they increased their physical activity to simulate mania. Physical activity increased 5-HIAA, but it is not clear that this was due to increased serotonin turnover or to mixing of CSF from higher regions, which contain higher levels of 5-HIAA, with lumbar CSF (or to a combination of both mechanisms).

Nonetheless, this finding stimulated many animal studies on the effects of exercise. For example, Chaouloff and colleagues showed that exercise increased tryptophan and 5-HIAA in rat ventricles. More recent studies using intra-cerebral dialysis have shown that exercise increases extracellular serotonin and 5-HIAA in various brain areas, including the hippocampus and cortex.

Two different mechanisms may be involved in this effect. As reviewed by Jacobs and Fornal, motor activity increases the firing rates of serotonin neurons, and these results in increased release and synthesis of serotonin.

In addition, there is an increase in the brain of the serotonin precursor tryptophan that persists after exercise.

The largest body of work in humans looking at the effect of exercise on tryptophan availability to the brain is concerned with the hypothesis that fatigue during exercise is associated with elevated brain tryptophan and serotonin synthesis.

A large body of evidence supports the idea that exercise, including exercise to fatigue, is associated with an increase in plasma tryptophan and a decrease in the plasma level of the branched chain amino acids (BCAAs) leucine, isoleucine and valine. The BCAAs inhibit tryptophan transport into the brain.

Because of the increase in plasma tryptophan and decrease in BCAA, there is a substantial increase in tryptophan availability to the brain. Tryptophan is an effective mild hypnotic, a fact that stimulated the hypothesis that it may be involved in fatigue.

The conclusion of these studies is that, in humans, a rise in precursor availability should increase serotonin synthesis during and after exercise and that this is not related to fatigue, although it may be related to improved mood. Whether motor activity increases the firing rate of serotonin neurons in humans, as in animals, is not known. However, it is clear that aerobic exercise can improve mood.

As with exposure to bright light, there has been a large change in the level of vigorous physical exercise experienced since humans were hunter-gatherers or engaged primarily in agriculture.

Lambert argued that the decline in vigorous physical exercise and, in particular, in effort-based rewards may contribute to the high level of depression in today's society. The effect of exercise on serotonin suggests that the exercise itself, not the rewards that stem from exercise, may be important.

If trials of exercise to prevent depression are successful, then prevention of depression can be added to the numerous other benefits of exercise.

The most important factor that could play a role in raising brain serotonin is diet. According to some evidence, tryptophan, which increases brain serotonin in humans as in experimental animals, is an effective antidepressant in mild-to-moderate depression. Further, in healthy people with high trait irritability, it increases agreeableness, decreases depression and improves mood.

However, whether tryptophan should be considered primarily as a drug or a dietary component is a matter of some dispute. In the United States, it is classified as a dietary component, but Canada and some European countries classify it as a drug.

Treating tryptophan as a drug is reasonable because, first, there is normally no situation in which purified tryptophan is needed for dietary reasons, and second, purified tryptophan and foods containing tryptophan have different effects on brain serotonin.

Although purified tryptophan increases brain serotonin, foods containing tryptophan do not. This is because tryptophan is transported into the brain by a transport system that is active toward all the large neutral amino acids and tryptophan is the least abundant amino acid in protein.

There is competition between the various amino acids for the transport system, so after the ingestion of a meal containing protein, the rise in the plasma level of the other large neutral amino acids will prevent the rise in plasma tryptophan from increasing brain tryptophan.

α-Lactalbumin, a minor constituent of milk, is one protein that contains relatively more tryptophan than most proteins.

Acute ingestion of α-lactalbumin by humans can improve mood and cognition in some circumstances, presumably owing to increased serotonin. Enhancing the tryptophan content of the diet chronically with α-lactalbumin is probably not practical.

However, increasing the tryptophan content of the diet relative to that of the other amino acids is something that possibly occurred in the past and could occur again in the future. Kerem and colleagues studied the tryptophan content of both wild chickpeas and the domesticated chickpeas that were bred from them in the Near East in Neolithic times.

The mean protein content (per mg dry seed) was similar for 73 cultivars and 15 wild varieties.

In the cultivated group, however, the tryptophan content was almost twice that of the wild seeds. Interestingly, the greater part of the increase was due to an increase in the free tryptophan content

In cultivated chickpeas, almost two-thirds of the tryptophan was in the free form.

Kerem and colleagues argue that there was probably selection for seeds with higher tryptophan content. This is plausible, given another example of an early strategy to increase the available tryptophan content of an important food source. Pellagra is a disorder caused by niacin deficiency, usually owing to poverty and a diet relying heavily on corn which has a low level of niacin and its precursor tryptophan.

Cultures in the Americas that relied greatly on corn used alkali during its processing (e.g., boiling the corn in lime when making tortillas). This enhanced the nutritional quality of the corn by increasing the bioavailability of both niacin and tryptophan, a practice that prevented pellagra.

The Europeans transported corn around the world but did not transport the traditional alkali-processing methods, thereby causing epidemics of pellagra in past centuries.

Breeding corn with higher tryptophan content was shown in the 1980s to prevent pellagra; presumably, it also raised brain serotonin.

In a recent issue of *Nature Biotechnology*, Morris and Sands argue that plant breeders should be focusing more on nutrition than on yield.

They ask, "Could consumption of tryptophan-rich foods play a role in reducing the prevalence of depression and aggression in society?"

Cross-national studies have reported a positive association between corn consumption and homicide rates and a negative association between dietary tryptophan and suicide rates. A

The idea behind such studies is interesting, any causal attribution must remain speculative, given the possible confounds.

Nonetheless, the possibility that the mental health of a population could be improved by increasing the dietary intake of tryptophan relative to the dietary intake of other amino acids remains an interesting idea that should be explored.

The effect of non-pharmacologic interventions on brain serotonin and the implications of increased serotonin for mood and behaviour need to be studied more.

The amount of money and effort put into research on drugs that alter serotonin is very much greater than that put into non-pharmacologic methods. The magnitude of the discrepancy is probably neither in tune with the wishes of the public nor optimal for progress in the prevention and treatment of mental disorders.

Serotonin isn't found in foods, but tryptophan is. Foods high in protein, iron, riboflavin, and vitamin B6 all tend to contain large amounts of the amino acid. Unfortunately, though, boosting your serotonin levels isn't as simple as eating a "high tryptophan diet."

Carbs cause the body to release more insulin, which promotes amino acid absorption and leaves tryptophan in the blood. If you mix high-tryptophan foods with carbs, you might get a serotonin boost

The tryptophan you find in food has to compete with other amino acids to be absorbed into the brain, so it's unlikely to have much of an effect on your serotonin levels. This differs from tryptophan supplements, which contain purified tryptophan and do have on serotonin levels.

While they can't compete with supplements — which you should not be taking without approval from your doctor — the foods listed below contain high amounts of tryptophan. Your best chance at achieving a serotonin boost without using supplements is to eat them often, with a serving of healthy carbohydrates, like rice, oatmeal, or whole-grain bread.

Eggs

Chicken eggs are the most commonly eaten eggs. They supply all essential amino acids for humans , a source of 'complete protein' and provide several vitamins and minerals as significant amounts of the Daily Value, including retinol (vitamin A), riboflavin, pantothenic acid, vitamin B12, choline and phosphorus.

A 100 gram serving of eggs provides 155 calories (kcal) of food energy and 12.6 g of protein. Vitamins A and D are in the egg yolk, one of the few foods to naturally contain vitamin D.

A yolk contains more than two-thirds of the recommended daily intake of 300 mg of cholesterol .

The yolk makes up about 33% of the liquid weight of the egg, containing all of the fat, slightly less than half of the protein, and most of the other nutrients.

More than half the calories found in eggs come from the fat in the yolk; 50 grams of chicken egg contains approximately 5 grams of fat. People on a low-cholesterol diet may need to reduce egg consumption; however, only 27% of the fat in egg is saturated fat.

The egg white consists primarily of water (87%) and protein (13%) and contains no cholesterol and little, if any, fat.

Harold McGee argues that the cholesterol in the yolk is not what causes a problem, because fat (in particular, saturated) is much more likely to raise cholesterol levels than the actual consumption of cholesterol.

The protein in eggs can significantly boost your blood plasma levels of tryptophan, according to recent research. For dinner, try making a simple baked egg, which you can easily combine or cook with leftovers. Or get fancy with this spinach-and-mushroom frittata. Don't leave out the yolks! They're extremely rich in both tryptophan and tyrosine, which are major contributors to the antioxidant properties of eggs.

Baked eggs make a tidy little meal, especially when served with fruit and a slice of whole grain toast.

They are also a surprisingly versatile vehicle for leftovers. For example, you could replace the tomato, spinach, basil, and turkey bacon in this recipe with a scoop of leftover chili, curry, vegetable stew, or beans and rice

You will need :

1 slice of tomato,

$\frac{1}{4}$ cup of baby spinach, rinsed and chopped

4 leaves of fresh basil, rinsed and chopped

1 piece turkey bacon or breast, chopped

1 large egg

Preheat your toaster oven to 180°C. Spray a ramekin or small oven-proof dish with low-fat cooking spray.

Place the tomato on the bottom of the dish, pack the spinach and basil on top, and arrange the turkey bacon over the greens. Crack the egg over the turkey bacon and garnish with freshly ground black pepper. Bake the egg for approximately 15 minutes – or until the yolk has set. Start checking your egg after 10 minutes or so, since the cooking time can vary from one toaster oven to another.

Baby Spinach and Mushroom Frittata is a perfect dish if you are watching your cholesterol.

You will need:

1 tsp minced garlic

1 medium onion

½ pound fresh mushrooms, chopped

1 tsp fresh rosemary

10-ounce bag fresh baby spinach, chopped

1 tbsp water

3 eggs

½ tsp black pepper

¼ crumbled goat cheese

Preheat oven to 180°C and spray a 10-inch nonstick, ovenproof skillet with cooking spray and place over medium-high heat.

When hot, sauté onion and garlic until onion is tender but not browned, about 5 minutes. Add mushrooms and rosemary and cook 5 minutes more. Add spinach and cook, turning constantly with tongs, until spinach completely wilts, about 3 minutes. Remove from heat and cool slightly. In a large bowl, beat together eggs and pepper. Stir in the spinach, mushroom mixture and goat cheese. Clean skillet and spray with cooking spray before returning to medium heat. When skillet is hot add egg mixture. Stir constantly for 1 minute then bake, uncovered, until set, 15 to 20 minutes.

Let frittata rest 5 minutes before inverting onto a large serving platter. Cut into 6 wedges. Serve hot or warm.

Cheese

Cheese is a food derived from milk that is produced in a wide range of flavours, textures, and forms by coagulation of the milk protein casein.

It comprises proteins and fat from milk, usually the milk of cows, buffalo, goats, or sheep. During production, the milk is usually acidified, and adding the enzyme rennet causes coagulation. The solids are separated and pressed into final form.

For a few cheeses, the milk is curdled by adding acids such as vinegar or lemon juice. Most cheeses are acidified to a lesser degree by bacteria, which turn milk sugars into lactic acid, then the addition of rennet completes the curdling.

Cheese is valued for its portability, long life, and high content of fat, protein, calcium, and phosphorus.

Cheese is more compact and has a longer shelf life than milk, although how long a cheese will keep depends on the type of cheese; labels on packets of cheese often claim that a cheese should be consumed within three to five days of opening. Generally speaking, hard cheeses, such as parmesan last longer than soft cheeses, such as Brie or goat's milk cheese.

The nutritional value of cheese varies widely.

Cottage cheese may consist of 4% fat and 11% protein; some whey cheeses 15% fat and 11% protein, and some triple-crème cheeses 36% fat and 7% protein. In general, cheese supplies a great deal of calcium, protein, phosphorus and fat.

A 30-gram (1.1 oz) serving of Cheddar cheese contains about 7 grams (0.25 oz) of protein and 200 milligrams of calcium.

Nutritionally, cheese is essentially concentrated milk: it takes about 200 grams (7.1 oz) of milk to provide that much protein, and 150 grams (5.3 oz) to equal the calcium.

Cheese is another great source of tryptophan. This classic macaroni recipe combines cheddar cheese with eggs and milk, which are also good sources of tryptophan.

For the **Classic Mac&Cheese** you will need:

8 ounces uncooked elbow macaroni

2 cups shredded sharp Cheddar cheese

1/2 cup grated Parmesan cheese

3 cups milk

1/4 cup butter

2 1/2 tablespoons all-purpose flour

2 tablespoons butter

1/2 cup bread crumbs

Cook macaroni according to the package directions then drain.

In a saucepan, melt butter or margarine over medium heat. Stir in enough flour to make a roux. Add milk to roux slowly, stirring constantly. Stir in cheeses, and cook over low heat until cheese is melted and the sauce is a little thick. Put macaroni in large casserole dish, and pour sauce over macaroni. Stir well.

Melt butter or margarine in a skillet over medium heat. Add breadcrumbs and brown. Spread over the macaroni and cheese to cover. Sprinkle with a little paprika.

Pineapples

The pineapple (Ananascomosus) is a tropical plant with edible multiple fruit consisting of coalesced berries, also called pineapples, and the most economically significant plant in the Bromeliaceae family.

Pineapples may be cultivated from a crown cutting of the fruit, possibly flowering in 20–24 months and fruiting in the following six months. Pineapple does not ripen significantly post-harvest

Pineapples can be consumed fresh, cooked, juiced, or preserved. They are found in a wide array of cuisines. In addition to consumption, the pineapple leaves are used to produce the textile . The fibres is also used as a component for wallpaper and other furnishings.

In a 100 gram serving, raw pineapple is an excellent source of manganese (44% Daily Value (DV)) and vitamin C (58% DV), but otherwise contains no essential nutrients in significant content .

Pineapples are a major source of bromelain, a protein that can reduce the side effects of chemotherapy as well as help suppress coughs, according to some research. Combine pineapples and coconut with chicken for this delicious piña colada chicken recipe.

Present in all parts of the pineapple plant, bromelain is a mixture of proteolytic enzymes. Bromelain is under preliminary research for a variety of clinical disorders, but to date has not been adequately defined for its effects in the human body. Bromelain may be unsafe for some users, such as in pregnancy, allergies, or anticoagulation therapy.

If having sufficient bromelain content, raw pineapple juice may be useful as a meat marinade and tenderizer.

Piña Colada Chicken is one way to mix the benefits of Bromelain with the fantastic taste of grill chicken.

Once you place the chicken on the grill, don't be tempted to turn it over. By having the bones facing the heat, the meat will remain juicy and tender.

You will need:

1 cup coconut milk

1 cup pineapple juice

1/4 cup lime juice

1 (4-pound) whole chicken

Whisk together first 3 ingredients and place in a large shallow dish. Using heavy-duty kitchen shears, cut chicken along both sides of the backbone.

Remove and discard backbone. Pull cut ends apart, and press to flatten chicken. Place in a dish with coconut-milk mixture, turning to coat.

Let stand at room temperature 30 minutes. DO NOT marinate longer as the pineapple juice will start to dissolve the meat.

Prepare grill for medium direct-heat cooking. Remove chicken from marinade; discard marinade. Pat chicken dry with paper towels.

Grill chicken, skin side up and covered with grill lid, 55 to 60 minutes or until thermometer registers 80 degrees C in the thickest portion of the thigh.

Remove from grill, and let stand 10 minutes before cutting.

Tofu

Tofu, also known as bean curd, is a food made by coagulating soy milk and then pressing the resulting curds into soft white blocks. It is a component in East Asian and Southeast Asian cuisines. There are many different varieties of tofu, including fresh tofu and tofu that has been processed in some way. Tofu is bought or made to be soft, firm, or extra firm. Tofu has a subtle flavour and can be used in savoury and sweet dishes. It is often seasoned or marinated to suit the dish.

Tofu originated in Han dynasty China some 2,000 years ago. Chinese legend ascribes its invention to prince Liu An (179-122 BC).

Tofu and its production technique were introduced into Korea and then Japan during the Nara period (710-794). Some scholars believe tofu arrived in Vietnam during the 10th and 11th century.

It spread into other parts of Southeast Asia as well. This spread probably coincided with the spread of Buddhism because it is an important source of protein in the vegetarian diet of East Asian Buddhism.

Li Shizhen in the Ming Dynasty described a method of making tofu in the Compendium of Materia Medica.

Tofu has a low calorie count and relatively large amounts of protein.

It is high in iron, and depending on the coagulants used in manufacturing (e.g. calcium chloride, calcium sulphate, magnesium sulphate), it can have higher calcium or magnesium content.

Tofu is considered a cool agent in Traditional Chinese medicine. It is claimed to invigorate the spleen, replenish qi, moisture and cool off Yang vacuity, and to detoxify the body.

In Chinese traditional medicine, tofu is suitable for those who are weak, malnourished, deficient in blood and qi; is suitable for old, slim or otherwise; suitable for those with high fat content in blood, high cholesterol, overweight, and with hardened blood vessels; suitable for people with diabetes; for mothers with low breast milk supply; for children and young adults; for those with inflamed respiratory tract, with phlegm, coughing and asthma. Tofu is also suited for people of old age; it is recommended to eat with liquor, since tofu contains cysteine, which can speed up the detoxification of alcohol in the body, and lessen the harm done to the liver, protecting the liver.

Tofu is relatively high in protein, about 10.7% for firm tofu and 5.3% for soft "silken" tofu with about 5% and 2% fat respectively as a percentage of weight.

In 1995, a report from the University of Kentucky, financed by Solae, concluded that soy protein is correlated with significant decreases in serum cholesterol, Low Density Lipoprotein LDL ("bad cholesterol") and triglyceride concentrations.

On the basis of this research, PTI, in 1998, filed a petition with Food and Drug Administration for a health claim that soy protein may reduce cholesterol and the risk of heart disease.

The FDA granted this health claim for soy: "25 grams of soy protein a day, as part of a diet low in saturated fat and cholesterol, may reduce the risk of heart disease." For reference, 100 grams of firm tofu coagulated with calcium sulphate contains 8.19 grams of soy protein.

Soy products are rich sources of tryptophan. You can substitute tofu for pretty much any protein, in pretty much any recipe, making it an excellent source of tryptophan for vegetarians and vegans.

Try these tofu vegetable kebabs, and reap the benefits of other ingredients like ginger and vitamin C-rich bell peppers.

Tofu Vegetable Kebabs: If you haven't tried tofu yet, it's time that you did! The USDA's MyPlate guide encourages diners to enjoy a wide variety of lean proteins, and tofu fits the bill.

It's low in fat, free of cholesterol, and wonderfully delicious when seasoned with a punchy Asian marinade.

You will need:

2 Tbsp. soy sauce

2 Tbsp. lemon juice

$\frac{1}{2}$ tsp. dry mustard

$\frac{1}{4}$ tsp. ground ginger

1 Tbsp. vegetable oil

1 package extra-firm tofu, rinsed, drained, and cut into 1-inch squares

1 medium red onion, peeled and cut into 1-inch squares

1 medium red bell pepper, seeded and cut into 1-inch squares

8 white mushrooms

Combine the soy sauce, lemon juice, mustard, and ginger. Add the vegetable oil in a slow and steady stream, whisking continuously. Add the tofu and toss to coat. Cover and refrigerate for at least two hours, tossing occasionally.

Thread the tofu and vegetables onto metal or wooden skewers, alternating pieces of tofu, onion, pepper, and mushrooms. Spray with non-stick cooking spray.

Grill the tofu and vegetable skewers over medium heat until tender (about 5-8 minutes), turning occasionally to ensure even cooking.

Salmon

Salmon is a popular food. Classified as an oily fish, salmon is considered to be healthy due to the fish's high protein, high omega-3 fatty acids, and high vitamin D content. Salmon is also a source of cholesterol, with a range of 23-214 mg/100 g depending on the species. According to reports in the journal Science, however, farmed salmon may contain high levels of dioxins. PCB levels may be up to eight times higher in farmed salmon than in wild salmon, but still far below levels considered dangerous.

Nonetheless, according to a 2006 study published in the Journal of the American Medical Association, the benefits of eating even farmed salmon far outweigh any risks imposed by contaminants

A simple rule of thumb is that the vast majority of Atlantic salmon available on the world market are farmed (almost 99%), whereas the majority of Pacific salmon are wild caught (greater than 80%).

Canned salmon in the U.S. is usually wild Pacific catch, though some farmed salmon is available in canned form. Smoked salmon is another popular preparation method, and can either be hot or cold smoked. Lox can refer either to cold smoked salmon or to salmon cured in a brine solution (also called gravlax).

Traditional canned salmon includes some skin (which is harmless) and bone (which adds calcium). Skinless and boneless canned salmon is also available.

Ordinary types of cooked salmon contain 500-1500 mg DHA and 300-1000 mg EPA per 100 grams.

Unlike most common farmed fish, bones of salmon are not easy to notice in the mouth because they are usually quite thin and not tough.

It's hard to go wrong with salmon, which, as you may have guessed, is also rich in tryptophan. Follow this recipe and steam it with lemony zucchini, bake it with asparagus and crumbled feta, or go crazy on the tryptophan rush and combine it with eggs and milk to make a smoked salmon frittata!

Seared Salmon with Zucchini (Courgettes) Lemon-Thyme Noodles

Ready to try a tasty new dish? We hope you're looking forward to putting salmon on the menu tonight.

You will need:

8 ounces spaghetti or fettuccini

1 pound salmon fillet

1/4 teaspoon salt

1/4 teaspoon freshly ground pepper

2 medium zucchini(Courgettes), shredded

2 tablespoons fresh lemon juice

1 teaspoon fresh thyme leaves, or 1/2 teaspoon dried

Cook pasta according to package directions.

Meanwhile, cut salmon into 1-inch slices and sprinkle with salt and pepper. Cook salmon, over medium-high heat, in a large non-stick sauté pan sprayed with cooking spray, 1 minute on each side or until desired degree of doneness. Remove and set aside.

Return sauté pan to medium heat and add zucchini, lemon juice and thyme. Cook, stirring gently, 2 to 3 minutes or until zucchini is just tender. Add drained pasta and toss to combine. Serve salmon on top of pasta.

Salmon and Asparagus enPapillote.

This refreshing recipe features a great mix of fish, asparagus, lemon, and crumbled feta.

You will need:

4 (18- x 12-inch) pieces aluminium foil

4(6 oz.) salmon filets

1/2 tsp. salt

1/4 tsp. freshly ground pepper

1 lemon, thinly sliced

4 sprigs fresh dill

1 lb. asparagus

1/2 cup grape tomatoes, halved

1/4 cup crumbled feta

Preheat oven to 240°C . Place foil pieces evenly over a large rimmed baking sheet.

Sprinkle salmon filets evenly with salt and pepper and place in centre of foil sheets.

Break off tough ends of asparagus and cut into 3-inch pieces. Layer lemon slices and dill over fish; sprinkle asparagus, tomatoes, and feta evenly over centre of each filet.

Fold into 1-inch folds the 2 long sides of foil sheets, sealing ends to form a packet, leaving a 2-inch space from fish (for heat to circulate inside packet).Bake for 15 minutes. Remove from oven and let stand 3 minutes; carefully open packets before serving.

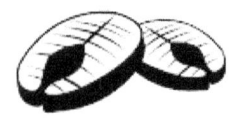

Smoked Salmon Frittata .Frittatas are great for breakfast, brunch, or a light dinner.

Ingredients:

1 tablespoon olive oil

1/2 cup chopped red onion

4 ounces smoked salmon, roughly chopped

1 tablespoon capers

3 eggs

1/4 cup 2% milk

1/4 teaspoon sea salt

1/4 teaspoon freshly cracked black pepper

1 (3-ounce) package cream cheese, cubed

1 tablespoon chopped chives

Preheat the oven to 180°C.Heat olive oil in an 8-inch oven-proof sauté pan over medium heat.

Add onion and cook until translucent but not brown, about 4 minutes. Add the salmon and capers and cook 1 minute, stirring occasionally.

Whisk eggs, milk, salt, and pepper until well beaten. Pour over salmon and stir gently with a rubber spatula, 30 seconds. Scatter cream cheese over the top and cook, without stirring, until the edges appear firm, about 3 minutes.

Transfer skillet to oven and bake until nicely browned and puffed, about 20 minutes.

To serve, invert onto a serving plate, cut into wedges and top with chopped chives.

Nuts and Seeds

We've all been there: It's 2 p.m. and you're hungry. Next time you feel like falling victim to those sugar, salt, and carbohydrate-filled choices, reach for a handful of nuts instead! Nuts are small but mighty nutritional powerhouses that are full of flavour. They contain protein, fibres, vitamins, minerals, antioxidants, and healthy (unsaturated) fats, all of which promote various aspects of health.

Almonds are a great choice for those looking to feel more full. They are high in protein (30.2 grams per cup), fibres (17.9 grams per serving), and fat (71.4 grams per serving). Almonds also contain the highest amount of calcium per serving (385 mg) of all nuts. Try adding sliced almonds to your salad for extra crunch!

Pistachios. If you want to promote your heart health, pistachios are a delicious way to do it. Not only are they low in sodium (only 1 mg), they contain potassium (1261 mg) and magnesium (149 mg), which can help control your blood pressure. They also contain a good amount of calcium (129 mg). With 24.9 grams of protein and 12.7 grams of fibres, you can feel good about adding these colourful nuts to a wide variety of meals.

Walnuts. In addition to being an excellent source of heart-healthy omega-3 fatty acids, walnuts can help fight fatigue! A cup of walnut pieces contains 18.3 grams of protein, and when added to an unrefined carbohydrate like oatmeal or leafy greens, they can help give you the energy you need.

Brazil Nuts. Along with walnuts, Brazil nuts are a great source of omega-3 fatty acids. With only 1 mg of sodium per serving, they are a great choice if you're watching your cholesterol. One serving contains 160 mg of magnesium and 280 mg of potassium, which both promote heart health and keep blood pressure in check. They're also a great source of selenium, which can help keep arthritis symptoms in check.

Hazelnuts. Are you an expecting mother? If so, consider incorporating hazelnuts into your diet. Hazelnuts rank highest among nuts when it comes to folate (153 mg per cup), which is a vitamin known to decrease the risk of birth defects. While it may be tempting to just reach for the Nutella, opt for a healthier option like adding chopped, toasted hazelnuts to a warm orange salad.

Cashews are more carbohydrate-rich than other nuts, and one ounce contains about 1.8 mg of iron, which makes them an ideal choice for athletes. They are also a good source of protein (5.2 g) and zinc (1.6 mg per serving), nutrients that play a critical role in cell growth and repair. Cashew butter is a great alternative to peanut butter; spread 2 tablespoons over a piece of whole grain bread.

Pecans. Not only do pecans contain more healthy fats than most other nuts, they're also a good source of fibres (9.5 grams per cup of pecan halves) and potassium (406 mg). They also contain arginine, an amino acid linked to good heart health.

Peanuts. Okay, so peanuts are not actually nuts. They're technically legumes. However, they share many of the same health benefits as nuts. They're an excellent source of protein, with 37.7 grams per cup. They also contain a lot of fibres (12.4 grams), magnesium (245 mg), and potassium (1029 mg). Peanut butter is a great addition to a smoothie; check out this peanut butter banana smoothie recipe!

Pine nuts are rich in healthy fats, and are a good source of many vitamins and minerals, specifically iron. One cup contains 7.5 grams of iron. Pine nuts also have high amounts of phosphorus (776 mg) and potassium (806 mg). Use them to make your own pesto at home, or add some toasted pine nuts to a green salad!

With so many crunchy, flavours-filled options, isn't it time you got a little nutty? Pick and choose your favourites , because all nuts and seeds contain tryptophan. Studies show that eating a handful of nuts a day can lower your risk for cancer, heart disease, and respiratory problems. They're also good sources of fibres, vitamins, and antioxidants.

For a nutty dinner, try the almond couscous. Or just go straight for dessert with some no-bake oatmeal peanut butter cookies.

Almond Couscous is a simple and very nutritious dish to prepare. And toasting the almonds adds a tremendous amount of flavour, so don't be tempted to skip it! Toasting the almonds adds a tremendous amount of flavour. Simply put the almonds in a 180 C oven when the couscous is resting for 5 minutes. By the time the couscous is ready, your almonds will be toasted.

Ingredients:
1 1/2 cups vegetable or chicken stock
2 teaspoons ground turmeric
1/4 to 1/2 teaspoon red pepper flakes
1 cup uncooked plain couscous
1/2 cup dried cranberries
1/2 cup toasted sliced almonds

Combine stock, turmeric and red pepper flakes in a large saucepan. Bring mixture to a boil over high heat. Stir in couscous and cranberries, cover and let stand 5 minutes. Add almonds and fluff mixture with a fork to combine. Serve immediately.

No-Bake Peanut Butter Oatmeal Cookies.

These no-bake cookies are perfect for when you want a little something healthy in a hurry.

Ingredients:
3 tablespoons skim milk
1/3 cup sugar
1 tablespoon cocoa powder
$1\frac{1}{2}$ teaspoons vanilla
1/3 cup crunchy peanut butter
1 cup quick-cooking oatmeal
2 tablespoons wheat germ

In a large saucepan, whisk together milk, sugar and cocoa and bring to a boil over medium-high heat—making sure to whisk constantly. Remove from heat, add peanut butter and vanilla and stir until smooth. Add oatmeal and wheat germ. Stir vigorously to combine. Drop by heaping tablespoons onto parchment paper and allow setting for at least one hour. One cookie will have just 98 calories and no cholesterol.

Turkey

Turkeys are sold sliced and ground, as well as "whole" in a manner similar to chicken with the head, feet, and feathers removed.

Frozen whole turkeys remain popular. Sliced turkey is frequently used as a sandwich meat or served as cold cuts; in some cases where recipes call for chicken it can be used as a substitute.

Ground turkey is sold just as ground beef, and is frequently marketed as a healthy alternative to beef. Without careful preparation, cooked turkey is usually considered to end up less moist than other poultry meats such as chicken or duck.

Wild turkeys, while technically the same species as domesticated turkeys, have a very different taste from farm-raised turkeys. Almost all of the meat is "dark" (even the breast) with a more intense flavour. The flavour can also vary seasonally with changes in available forage, often leaving wild turkey meat with a gamier flavour in late summer due to the greater number of insects in its diet over the preceding months. Wild turkey that has fed predominantly on grass and grain has a milder flavour. Older heritage breeds also differ in flavour.

A large amount of turkey meat is processed. It can be smoked and as such is sometimes sold as turkey ham or turkey bacon, which is widely considered to be far healthier than pork-based bacon.

Twisted helices of deep fried turkey meat, sold as "turkey twizzlers", came to prominence in the UK in 2004 when chef Jamie Oliver campaigned to have them and similar foods removed from school dinners.

Turkeys are traditionally eaten as the main course of Thanksgiving in the United States and Canada, and at Christmas feasts in much of the rest of the world (often as stuffed turkey). It was eaten as such as early as the 16th century in England.

Before the 20th century, pork ribs were the most common food for the North American holidays, as the animals were usually slaughtered in November. Turkeys were once so abundant in the wild that they were eaten throughout the year, the food considered commonplace, whereas pork ribs were rarely available outside of the Thanksgiving-New Year season,

While the tradition of turkey at Christmas spread throughout England in the 17th century among the working classes it became common to serve goose, which remained the predominant roast until the Victorian era.

In the UK in 2009, 7,734,000 turkeys were consumed on Christmas Day.

Roast turkey :Both fresh and frozen turkeys are used for cooking; as with most foods, fresh turkeys are generally preferred, although they cost more. Around holiday seasons, high demand for fresh turkeys often makes them difficult to purchase without ordering in advance. For the frozen variety, the large size of the turkeys typically used for consumption makes defrosting them a major endeavour: a typically sized turkey will take several days to properly defrost.

Turkeys are usually baked or roasted in an oven for several hours, often while the cook prepares the remainder of the meal.

Sometimes, a turkey is brined before roasting to enhance flavour and moisture content. This is necessary because the dark meat requires a higher temperature to denature all of the myoglobin pigment than the white meat (very low in myoglobin), so that fully cooking the dark meat tends to dry out the breast.

Brining makes it possible to fully cook the dark meat without drying the breast meat. Turkeys are sometimes decorated with turkey frills, paper frills or "booties" that are placed on the end of drumsticks or bones of other cutlets.

In some areas, particularly the American South, they may also be deep fried in hot oil (often peanut oil) for 30 to 45 minutes by using a turkey fryer.

Deep frying turkey has become something of a fad, with hazardous consequences for those unprepared to safely handle the large quantities of hot oil required.

Turkey contains more protein per ounce than other meats. The white meat of turkey is generally considered healthier than dark meat because of its lower saturated fat content, but the nutritional differences are small.

Turkey is reputed to cause sleepiness, but holiday dinners are commonly large meals served with carbohydrates, fats, and alcohol in a relaxed atmosphere, all of which are bigger contributors to post-meal sleepiness than the tryptophan in turkey.

After World War II, cheap imported turkey tail became popular in Samoa.

Because the cut is so fatty, it has been attributed to the rise in obesity rates in the Pacific.

To combat obesity, turkey tails were banned from 2007 to 2013, only allowed back in Samoa to appease the demands of the World Trade Organization

There's a reason why the Thanksgiving meal is usually followed by a siesta on the couch — turkey is essentially stuffed tryptophan. Try this recipe for an Asian turkey rice bowl that's both tangy and healthy.

Turkey Rice Bowl. This marinade is very strong, so you don't have to marinate it too long: just 10 to 15 minutes at room temperature.

Ingredients:

1/3 cup hoisin sauce

2 tablespoons dark mushroom soy sauce

1 tablespoon mirin or dry white wine

1 teaspoon freshly grated ginger

1 teaspoon hot sauce

1 1/2 lbs turkey tenderloin

1 cup julienned snow peas

1 tablespoon vegetable oil

1 teaspoon toasted sesame oil

1 tablespoon toasted sesame seeds

4 cups hot cooked rice

Stir together first 5 ingredients. Pour 1/3 of mixture into a shallow dish. Slice tenderloins into 1&1/2 to 2-inch-thick pieces and place in shallow dish with the prepared sauce, turning to coat. Let stand at room temperature for 10 minutes.

Heat indoor or outdoor grill to medium-high. Remove turkey from the marinade, and discard marinade.

Pat turkey dry with paper towels. Place on grill grate and cook covered, 5 minutes per side, basting twice with reserved sauce. Remove from grill and let rest 5 minutes before slicing.

In a large skillet, heat vegetable and sesame oil over medium-high heat. Sauté snow peas, stirring constantly, 3 to 4 minutes or until crisp and tender. Serve turkey with snow peas and cooked rice.

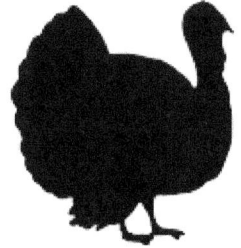

Positivity

Research shows that facing daily life and your interactions with others with a positive outlook can significantly boost your serotonin levels.

Dalai Lama said : ""Happiness is not something ready made. It comes from your own actions." and Aristotel added: ""Happiness is the meaning and the purpose of life, the whole aim and end of human existence."

And yet, this search for happiness can be a lifelong search, especially if we look at happiness as something that will come once we achieve certain goals, a nice home, a perfect spouse, the perfect job, and when we get these goals, instead of being happy, we often are looking forward to being happy when we meet our next goals.

Life shouldn't be an on-going chase for promotions and a hunger for material possessions, houses or expensive cars.

Happiness shouldn't be something that happens to us in the future, maybe someday, if things go well.

Happiness should be here and now, who we are now, with the people we're with now, doing the things we're doing now. And if we're not with people who make us happy, and doing things that make us happy then we should take action to make that happen.

Don't wait for happiness. Seize it. Follow Leo Tolstoy advice :"If you want to be happy, be."

Be present. Don't think about how great things will be in the future. Don't dwell on what did or didn't happen in the past.

Learn to be in the here and now, and experience life as it's happening, and appreciate the world for the beauty that it is, right now. Practice makes perfect with this crucial skill.

Connect with others. In my experience, very few things can achieve happiness as well as connecting with other human beings, cultivating relationships, bonding with others. Some tips on doing this.

Spend time with those you love. This might seem almost the same as the item above, and in reality it's an extension of the same concept, a more specific application. Spending time with the people you love is extremely important to happiness and yet it's incredible how often we do just the opposite, and spend time alone, or disconnected from those we love, or spend time with people we don't much like just to make money or a financial gain. Make it a priority to schedule time with the people you love. Make that your most important item of the day. I ensure my happiness by letting nothing come between me and the people I love most.

Do the things you love. What do you love doing most? Figure out the things you love doing most in life, the things that make you happiest, and make those the foundation of your day, every day. Eliminate as much of the rest as possible.

For me, the things I love doing are spending time with wife and my boy, refereeing, running and playing Poker, Hearthstone or World of Warcraft . I do those things every day, and very little else. It may take awhile to get your life down to your essentials like I have

Focus on the good things. Everyone's life has positive and negative aspects, whether you're happy or not depends largely on which aspects you focus on. Did you lose today's poker game? At least you got to spend time with friends doing something fun. Did you sprain your ankle running or you have a muscle ache ? Well, your body probably needed a week's rest anyway, as you were running too much! Did your baby get sick? Well, at least it's only a flu virus and nothing life-threatening and at least you have a wonderful baby to nurse to health!

You can see my point, almost everything has a positive side, and focusing on the positives make all the difference.

What piece of advice were they more adamant about than any other? More adamant about than lessons regarding marriage, children and happiness?

Do not stay in a job you dislike. You know those nightmares where you are shouting a warning but no sound comes out? Well, that's the intensity with which the experts wanted to tell younger people that spending years in a job you dislike is a recipe for regret and a tragic mistake. Take a lesson from people who have already seen most of what life has to offer: do not waste time in a job you hate.

Do work you love. An extension, of course, of doing the things you love, but applied to work. Are you already doing the work you love? Then you're one of the lucky ones, and you should appreciate how lucky you are. If you aren't doing the work you love, you should make it a priority to try to find work you're passionate about, and to steer your career in that direction.

Take myself for example: I was doing work that I was good at but that I wasn't passionate about and the place I was working was draining me out and I was tired when I was doing my refereeing. I quit a full-time job, started a part-time job which is more enjoyable and focused on my football refereeing. Also was passionate

Find time for peace. With the hectic pace of life these days, it's hard to find a moment of peace. But if you can make time for solitude and quiet, it can be one of the happiest parts of your day. Here's how.

Notice the small things. Instead of waiting for the big things to happen , marriage, kids, house, nice car, big promotion, winning the lottery, find happiness in the small things that happen every day.

Little things like having a quiet cup of coffee in the early morning hours, or the delicious and simple taste of berries, or the pleasure of reading a book with your child, or taking a walk or a dinner in town with your partner. Noticing these small pleasures, throughout your day, makes a huge difference.

Develop compassion. Compassion is developing a sense of shared suffering with others and taking steps to alleviate the suffering of others.

I think too often we forget about the suffering of others while focusing on our own suffering, and if we learned to share the suffering of others, our suffering would seem insignificant as a result.

Compassion is an extremely valuable skill to learn, and you get better with practice. Here's how.

Be grateful. Learning to be grateful for what's in our lives, for the people who have enriched our lives, goes a long way toward happiness. It helps us to appreciate what we have and what we have received, and the people who have helped us. Read more.

Become a lifelong learner. I find an inordinate amount of pleasure in reading, in learning about new things, in enriching my knowledge as I get older. I think spending time reading some of the classics, as well as passionately pursuing new interests, is energy well invested. Try to do a little of it every day, and see if it doesn't make you happier.

Simplify your life. This is really about identifying the things you love and then eliminating everything else as much as possible. By simplifying your life in this way, you create time for your happiness, and you reduce the stress and chaos in your life. In my experience, living a very simple life is also a pleasure in itself.

Slow down. Similar to simplifying, slowing down is just a matter of reminding yourself that there's no need to rush through life. Schedule less things on your calendar, and more space between things. Even better then less things on your calendar is to throw the calendar. Don't to "To Do List" . Learn to eat slower, drive slower, walk slower. Going slowly helps to reduce stress, and improve the pleasure of doing things, and keeps you in the present moment.

Exercise. I've written about the pleasures of exercise many times. It can be hard to start an exercise program but once you get going, it relieves stress and can really give you a good feeling. I feel joyful every time I run.

Meditate. You don't need to join a Yoga course or get a mat or learn any lotus positions, but the simplest form of meditation can really help you to be present and to get out of the worrying part of your head. You can do it right now: close your eyes and simply try to focus on your breathing as long as possible. Pay attention to the breath as it comes into your body, and then as it goes out. When you feel your mind start to wander, don't fret, but just simply acknowledge the other thoughts, and then return to your breathing. Do this a little each day and you'll get better at it.

Learn to accept. One of the challenges for people like me, people who want to improve themselves and change the world, is learning to accept things as they are. Sometimes it's better to learn to accept, and to love, the world as it is, and people as they are, rather than to try to make everything and everyone conform to an impossible ideal. I'm not saying you should accept cruelty and injustice, but learn to love things when they are less than "perfect".

Spend time in nature. Go outside and take a walk each day, or take the time to watch a sunset or sunrise. Or find a body of water, the ocean, a lake, a river, a pond — and spend time taking a look at it, contemplating it. If you're lucky enough to live near some woods, or a mountain, or a canyon, go hiking. Time in nature is time invested in your happiness. When I was a student in Galati I had the Danube in there. Every time when I was upset or my mood was low I was going at the river side and listen the water, listen to the wind, listen to the gulls in the sky.

This was my cure for sadness and had always worked.

Find the miracles in life. I absolutely believe in miracles, and believe that they are all around us, every day. My children are all miracles. The kindnesses of strangers are miracles. The life growing all around us is a miracle. Find those miracles in your life, and enjoy the majesty of them.

Some days I wake up with rocket fuel in my veins, ready to take the day by storm. Happiness comes totally natural. But on others it can feel like I have lead weights strapped to my shoes. The only way to feel better is to get rid of the weight, walk barefoot if needed.

Happiness is a practice. It's on us to learn it. While some days are easier to find a smile than others, happiness is a daily choice. It's a mind-set we can nurture and train. That doesn't mean it's there every second, but when you notice it's missing, often the tiniest shift can put you right back on top of the world.

Life will constantly test your ability to make a lemon martini out of the sourest of lemons. So be ready. Start strong. Do something first thing in the morning that will ensure your day is a success. This is the ace in the hole. It's easy to roll out of bed and onto the couch for some TV or into email for the rest of a meaningless day. You know this isn't the best way to wake up on top of the world. Wake up and go for a run, go do a breakfast in bed for your half, put a screw and repair that shelf which you said you will fix last month.

You know how good it feels to make progress on the meaningful things in your life. So do something about it. Write a poem or draw a picture.

Don't rush through tasks. One of the quickest creators of stress and killers of happiness is rushing and believing you don't have enough time to smell the roses. There is always time. And if you don't, the roses will eventually die.

Only plan to do one thing each day. Let the rest be a bonus. Plan twice as much time as you think it will take and don't fill every second of your calendar with tasks.

Humans are notorious for having ridiculous expectations of what we can get done in a day and how quickly things take. Hence we're left with a day full of stress and constant rushing. Speed alone can cause immediate stress.

If you always feel rushed, you'll never feel you have time to enjoy the subtle, non-task-related wonders of life. Do the above and you'll create space to be amazed by the world.

Walk in the sand with bare feet, play with a dog, feed a duck, go on a walk with no destination, catch a sunset, be in nature, or just find a bench and watch the world happen around you. Your pick.

When we are in an emotional state of pure gratitude, it's impossible to feel negative emotions like stress, anger, or unhappiness.

All of us have things that immediately change our state. That make us smile, get us inspired, and simply make us happy.

Maybe that's a special song, a movie, a YouTube cat video, a certain workout, a book, a drink or time with a friend. Keep track of these.

Smile. So simple yet so powerful. This is as contagious as it gets. Do it everywhere. Be known as the person who's always smiling, especially to those frowning. If someone is frustrated on the road or at a grocery store, just smile ear to ear. All it takes is a few people to reciprocate and it will spread exponentially. Plus all kinds of studies have shown that the physical act of smiling fires off chemicals in the brain that create happiness.

A nearly immediate route to happiness and fulfillment is to do something for someone else. It can be as simple as opening a door or as big as getting someone their dream job. This is what makes experiences rich. Do them daily. Be polite, say "Thank You!" , offer your sit in the bus to an old lady.

Caring about others is fundamental to our happiness. Helping other people is not only good for them; it's good for us too. It makes us happier and can help to improve our health. Giving also creates stronger connections between people and helps to build a happier society for everyone. It's not all about money - we can also give our time, ideas and energy. So if you want to feel good, do good.

Happiness not spent today does not equal more happiness tomorrow. For some, happiness comes easy. No thought or routine required. For others, simple reminders and practices are all it takes. Happiness is a choice. It always will be.

Happiness only exists today. There is no waiting. If you aren't happy today then you aren't happy. Don't convince yourself that some sacrifice today is worth the hope of happiness in the future.

We're constantly bombarded with messages about what makes for a good life. Advertisers tell us it comes from owning and consuming their products. The media associate it with wealth, beauty or fame. And politicians claim that nothing matters more than growing the economy. But do any of these things really bring lasting happiness?

For thousands of years, people have looked to philosophy, religion and grandmotherly wisdom for answers to such questions. But in recent decades this ancient wisdom has been tested by scientific research.

Scientists have found that although our genes and circumstances matter, a huge proportion of the variations in happiness between us come from our choices and activities.

So although we may not be able to change our inherited characteristics or the circumstances in which we find ourselves, we still have the power to change how happy we are - by the way we approach our lives.

Our relationships with other people are the most important thing for our happiness. People with strong relationships are happier, healthier and live longer.

Our close relationships with family and friends provide love, meaning, support and increase our feelings of self-worth. Our broader social networks bring a sense of belonging. So it's vital that we take action to strengthen our relationships and make new connections.

Our body and mind are connected. Being active makes us happier as well as healthier. It instantly improves our mood and can even lift us out of depression.

We don't all have to run marathons - there are simple things we can do to be more active each day.

We can also boost our wellbeing by spending time outdoors, eating healthily, unplugging from technology and getting enough sleep.

Be more active today. Get off the bus a stop early, take the stairs, turn off the TV, walk to the shop. Eat nutritious food, drink more water, catch up on sleep. Notice which healthy actions lift your mood and do more of them.

Have you ever felt there must be more to life? Good news, there is. And it's right here in front of us. We just need to stop and take notice. Learning to be more mindful and aware does wonders for our wellbeing, whether it's on our walk to work, in the way we eat or in our relationships. It helps us get in tune with our feelings and stops us dwelling on the past or worrying about the future.

Give yourself a bit of head space. At least once a day, stop and take five minutes to just breathe and be in the moment.

Notice and appreciate good things around you every day, big or small. Trees, birdsong, the smell of coffee, laughter perhaps?

Learning affects our wellbeing in lots of positive ways. It exposes us to new ideas and helps us stay curious and engaged. It also gives us a sense of accomplishment and helps boost our self-confidence and resilience. There are many ways to learn new things throughout our lives, not just through formal qualifications.

We can share a skill with friends, join a club, learn to sing, play a new sport and so much more.

Do something for the first time today. Sample sushi, sample a extra hot dish, try a cocktail ,try a new route, read a different newspaper or visit a local place of interest. Learn a new skill, however small. A first aid technique or a new feature on your phone, perhaps. Cook a new meal or use a new word.

Feeling good about the future is really important for our happiness. We all need goals to motivate us and these have to be challenging enough to excite us, but also achievable. If we try to attempt the impossible, this creates unnecessary stress. Choosing meaningful but realistic goals gives our lives direction and brings a sense of accomplishment and satisfaction when we achieve them.

All of us have times of stress, loss, failure or trauma in our lives. How we respond to these events has a big impact on our wellbeing. We often cannot choose what happens to us, but we can choose how we react to what happens. In practice it's not always easy, but one of the most exciting findings from recent research is that resilience, like many other life skills, can be learned.

Ask for help today. Confide in a friend, talk to an expert, reach out to a colleague, ask a neighbour to lend a hand. When something is troubling you, do something you really enjoy. Shift your mood and bring a new perspective on the problem.

Positive emotions, like joy, gratitude, contentment, inspiration and pride, don't just feel good when we experience them.

They also help us perform better, broaden our perception, increase our resilience and improve our physical health. So although we need to be realistic about life's ups and downs, it helps to focus on the good aspects of any situation – the glass half full rather than the glass half empty.

Nobody's perfect. But so often we compare a negative view of ourselves with an unrealistic view of other people. Dwelling on our flaws, what we're not rather than what we've got, makes it much harder to be happy. Learning to accept ourselves, warts and all, and being kinder to ourselves when things go wrong increases our enjoyment of life, our resilience and our wellbeing. It also helps us accept others as they are.

Be as kind to yourself as you are to others. See your mistakes as opportunities to learn. Notice things you do well, however small.

People who have meaning and purpose in their lives are happier, feel more in control and get more out of what they do. They also experience less stress, anxiety and depression. But where do we find meaning and purpose? It might come from doing a job that makes a difference, our religious or spiritual beliefs, or our family. The answers vary for each of us but they all involve being connected to something bigger than ourselves.

Feel part of something bigger. Spend time with children, visit an inspiring location, gaze at the stars or join a club. Be more charitable. Give others your time, offer to help neighbours or friends, consider giving blood or volunteering.

No one confuses the type of happiness ice cream brings with the positive feelings one gets from raising a good kid. Happiness is a vague word. We need happy feelings but we also need meaning in our lives.

And research shows they are related but distinct: Findings suggest that happiness is mainly about getting what one wants and needs, including from other people or even just by using money.

In contrast, meaningfulness was linked to doing things that express and reflect the self, and in particular to doing positive things for others. Meaningful involvements increase one's stress, worries, arguments, and anxiety, which reduce happiness.

Researchers at Tohoku University in Japan did a 7 year study of over 43,000 adults age 40 to 79 asking if they had ikigai (a Japanese term for meaning in life) and then tracked their health.

People with ikigai were much more likely to be alive 7 years later.

The lack of ikigai was in particular associated with death due to cardiovascular disease (usually stroke), but not death due to cancer.

Running marathons is painful. Completing them is awesome. Studying is boring. Having a degree feels great. Happiness in the moment is not everything.

In his TED talk, Daniel Kahneman, Nobel Prize winner and author of Thinking, Fast and Slow discussed two different types of happiness that sound very similar to the distinction between happiness and meaning.

The first is being happy in your life. It is happiness that you experience immediately and in the moment.

The second is being happy about your life. It is the happiness that exists in memory when we talk about the past and the big picture. Stories are key here. This is closer to 'meaning'.

There are also little easy tricks to feel good instantly:

Chill Out : Most people equate happiness with a sultry Caribbean beach or a Pina-Colada in Ibiza but a snowy mountain in Brasov may be more accurate. It turns out that cold temperatures can improve your mood. Researchers at the University of Michigan discovered that blowing cold air up participants' noses put them in a better frame of mind than did blasts of hot air. So if you need a boost, dial down the thermostat or go outside if is wintertime.

Remember Whence You Came: Don't underestimate the power of nostalgia. When you swap stories about the Prom night or the Christmas Marathon week with Valentin, Daniel and the others, you view yourself in a more positive light and form tighter bonds, says Dan Buettner, the author of Thrive: Finding Happiness the Blue Zones Way, a book about the happiest regions in the world. He also recommends "land-mining your home with photos and memorabilia, so you're constantly reminded of your history."

Don't Dwell. Mulling over past failures can be tempting, you feel as if you're gaining insights and finding answers), but over time this behaviour may lead to feelings of helplessness. Research shows that ruminators are more likely to be depressed, due to a downward spiral of emotions.

First you begin obsessing, which makes you lack the mental clarity to come up with potentially good solutions to problems; as a result, you lose confidence and feel unhappy, says Susan Nolen-Hoeksema, a professor of psychology at Yale University. So instead of going over something again and again, distract yourself with a movie or a game. Did you tried Hearthstone?

Spread the Wealth. Giving away money can make you happier than spending it on yourself, studies show. The same may be true of buying things for others rather than yourself.

Never borrow money to anyone.

Do little gift, buy a sandwich for a homeless, if you're going for coffee, take a colleague's order and foot the bill. Pick up a treat for a friend that you would normally impulse-buy for yourself at the checkout counter. And tip generously. The payoff will be yours.

Eat a Snack Around 2 p.m. That's when levels of serotonin, a brain chemical that helps regulate mood, can take a nosedive, according to Eric Braverman, a physician in New York City and the author of The Edge Effect. Ideally, choose one that contains mood-boosting nutritional powerhouses, like B vitamins (B6, B12, and folic acid, found in dairy products and leafy greens) and complex carbohydrates (try whole grains) or nuts and seeds.

Get a Move On ."For some people, exercising at high intensity three times a week for just 30 minutes at a time can provide the same benefits as some of the most powerful psychiatric medications," says psychologist Tal Ben-Shahar.

Research suggests that during that half hour of exercise, the human body can increase the production of a protein called brain-derived neurotrophic factor, which can have an antidepressant effect. Yoga, for its part, seems to have additional calming and happy-making effects on both the brain and the parasympathetic nervous system.

Limit Your Options. "When you make a choice, you generally want the best," says psychologist Barry Schwartz. "That means you tend to consider everything that's available, which can be overwhelming." Not to mention stressful and anxiety producing. Whenever you find yourself paralyzed by indecision, whether you're shopping for a new car, a new nail-polish colour, or a new jumper, quickly try to whittle down your options to a few choices. Then pick one and move on.

Learn a new skill. Start baking or learn to play golf. Or join a poker club. Just find something that occupies 100 percent of your attention while you're engaged in it. You'll be more motivated and focused —feelings that promote happiness, says Mihaly Csikszentmihalyi, a professor of psychology and management at Claremont Graduate University, in Claremont, California. Buettner says that in Denmark, characterized as the most thriving country in the world when it comes to well-being, according to a recently published Poll, a majority of the population reports belonging to a social club.

Make Your Bed. "When I was researching my book on happiness, this was the number one most impactful change that people brought up over and over," says author Gretchen Rubin.

Turns out, people are happier when everyday tasks in their lives are completed. And if hospital corners don't do it for you, test out other small ways to make your life more efficient and pleasant. Tidy up the shelves, put the shoes in order. Shoot for concrete changes: hanging a key hook in your entryway, finally moving your banking online or eating an yogurt each morning.

Lear to say "No" if you think accepting to do something will make you unhappy.

Remember you can't predict the future so you need to be happy today.

Be selfish in a good way, chose the people you love, the things you like, do what you enjoy and get rid of the people who keep you from progressing. They are the reason you are not as happy as you want.

Remember hope is not a strategy and having a boring life is bad for your health. Your health is always the most important aspect of your life and the easier way to improve health is to be happy.

Laughter is essential to our well-being and now is the moment when you need to create your own life.

This life is not the life others are telling you to have.

Be impeccable and always do your best, avoid regrets, don't do anything you don't want to do, be honest and don't make promises you can't keep.

Raise your Serotonin! Be Happy!

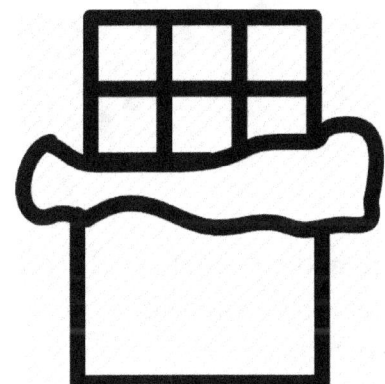

Chocolate is high in magnesium and other "feel good" nutrients.

Leafy Greans are energy enhancing

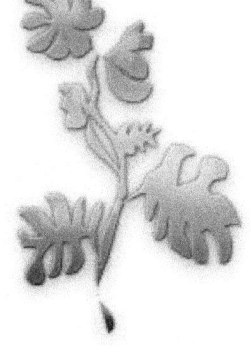

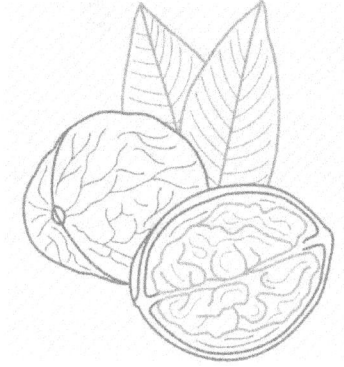

Walnuts are loaded with Omega 3 and other brain nutrients

Hot bath with salt helps calming

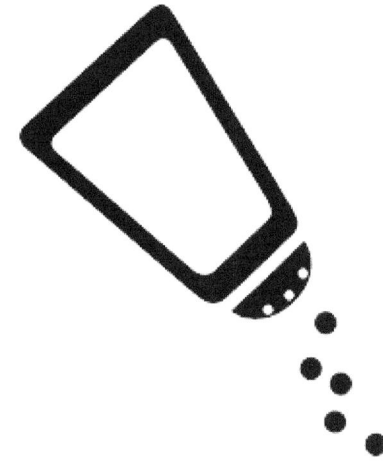

Water and a proper hydration increases energy and lowers stress

Cayenne peppers are the perfect depression relieve.

Bananas helps raise serotonin

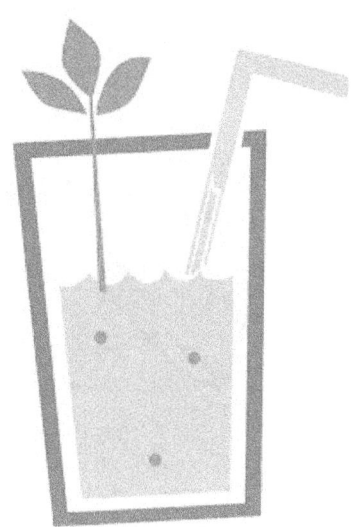

Green Smoothies are
an energy boost

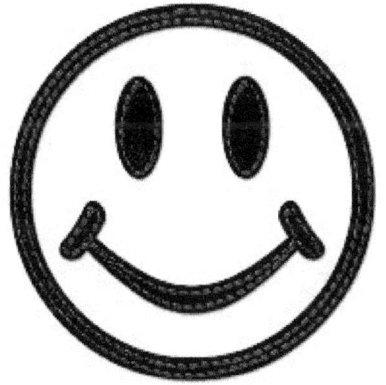

Smiling releases
happy hormones

Walking clears the mind
and raises serotonin

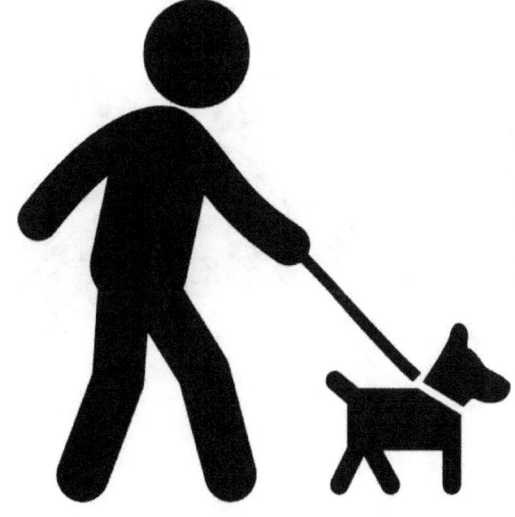

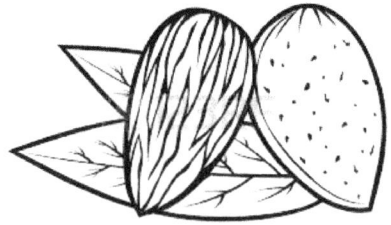 Almonds are brain food and are rich in magnesium

Oats eases depression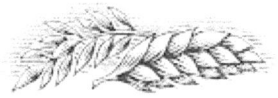

 Spending time in nature clears the mind and rise the serotonin level

Bibliography

1. Neumeister A, Young T, Stastny J. Implications of genetic research on the role of the serotonin in depression: emphasis on the serotonin type 1A receptor and the serotonin transporter.
2. Schoevers RA, Smit F, Deeg DJH, et al. Prevention of late-life depression in primary care: do we know where to begin?
3. Anguelova M, Benkelfat C, Turecki G. A systematic review of association studies investigating genes coding for serotonin receptors and the serotonin transporter: I. Affective disorders.
4. Kerem Z, Lev-Yadun S, Gopher A, et al. Chickpea domestication in the Neolithic Levant through the nutritional perspective.
5. Katz SH, Hediger ML, Valleroy LA. Traditional maize processing techniques in the new world: traditional alkali processing enhances the nutritional quality of the maize.
6. Xue-Cun C, Tai-An Y, Xiu-Zhen T, et al. Opaque-2 maize in the prevention and treatment of pellagra.
7. Voracek M, Tran US. Dietary tryptophan intake and suicide rate in industrialized nations.
8. https://en.wikipedia.org/wiki/Serotonin
9. http://www.medicalnewstoday.com/
10. http://www.healthline.com/
11. http://www.nhs.uk/

ABOUT THE AUTHOR

Paul Valentin Mihalache is a Romanian writer, born 04/06/1986, which lives in London, United Kingdom, since 2010.

With a Bachelor Degree in Physical Education and Sports and a PhD in Sports Activities he has dedicated his life and career to sport, especially to football.

He is a Level 4 FA Football Referee since 2014 , officiating in the United Counties Football League, Barclays U18 Premier League, Women's Super League and others Midlands and Bedfordshire Leagues.

The "Happiness Guide" is his second book and he wants to tackle the low-esteem generated by stress and other problems.

He invites all the readers to be happy.

www.ingramcontent.com/pod-product-compliance
Lightning Source LLC
Chambersburg PA
CBHW051344170526
45166CB00002B/957